Innovative Mediterranean Sea Diet Cooking Plan

Better Meals Thanks to These Mediterranean Recipes

Joseph Bellisario

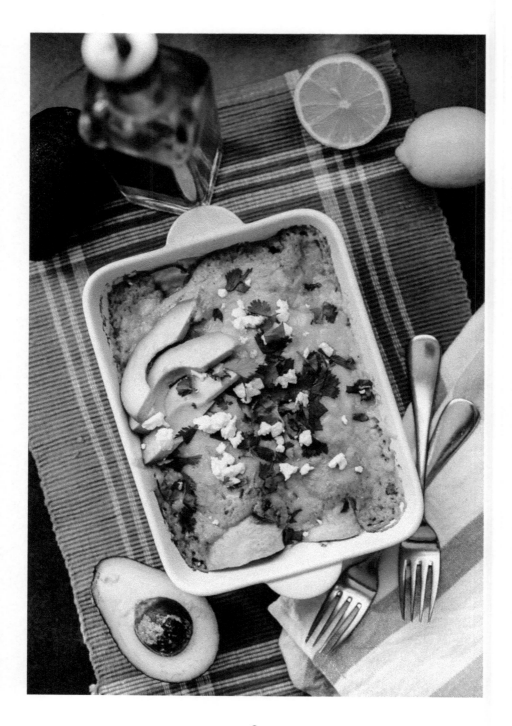

TABLE OF CONTENTS

5

Charred avocado an eggs

Ingredients

- ½ of a fresh red chili
- 4 spring onions
- A few sprigs of fresh soft herbs
- 2 tablespoons of cottage cheese
- ½ a ripe avocado
- Olive oil
- 1 sweet potato
- 1 red pepper
- 2 large free-range eggs

Directions

1. Heat 1 tablespoon of olive oil over a medium-high heat.
2. Add the spring onions together with the avocado and pepper, let fry for 4 minutes, or until lightly charred.
3. Add peeled potatoes to the pan, toss with the charred vegetables, let fry for 3 minutes.
4. Spread the vegetables evenly in the pan.
5. Dig out 2 pockets.
6. Crack an egg into each one, then tilt the pan so the whites run into the vegetables binding everything together.
7. Season with sea salt and black pepper.

8. Cover, with tin foil, lower the heat to medium–low, let the eggs cook for 5 minutes.
9. Spoon the mixture onto a plate, dollop with cottage cheese and sprinkle over the herbs.

Avocado and slow roasted tomatoes on the toast

Ingredients

- 4 handfuls of rocket
- 4 plum tomatoes
- 4 slices of sourdough bread
- Olive oil
- 150g of feta cheese
- 1 bunch of fresh basil
- 1 lemon
- 3 ripe avocados

Directions

1. Preheat the oven to 280°F.
2. Place the tomatoes cut-side up on a baking tray.
3. Season generously and drizzle with oil.
4. Then, roast gently for 2 hours or until dried out.
5. Pound basil leaves in a pestle and mortar with a pinch of sea salt until to foam paste.
6. Pour in a good splash of oil and squeeze in the juice of ½ lemon.

7. Place avocado flesh in a bowl, squeeze in the other lemon half.
8. Season with salt and pepper.
9. Mash with a fork to bring it all together.
10. Toast the bread, then divide between 4 plates and generously spread on the avocado and top with the tomatoes.
11. Serve and enjoy with crumbled feta.

Avocado ice cream

Ingredients

- 500ml of whole milk
- 200g of sugar
- 4 ripe avocados
- 2 vanilla pods
- 1 lime
- 1 lemon

Directions

1. Add vanilla to saucepan with the pods.
2. Add the sugar with the zest and juice.
3. Bring to the boil, let simmer for a couple of minutes to dissolve the sugar.
4. Remove from heat, pour into a bowl, let cool.
5. Once the syrup is cool, remove the vanilla pods.
6. Blend the avocado flesh with the milk to a smooth, light consistency.
7. Pour it into a large baking dish, place in a freezer.
8. Whisk every half hour or so until frozen and smooth.
9. Serve and enjoy.

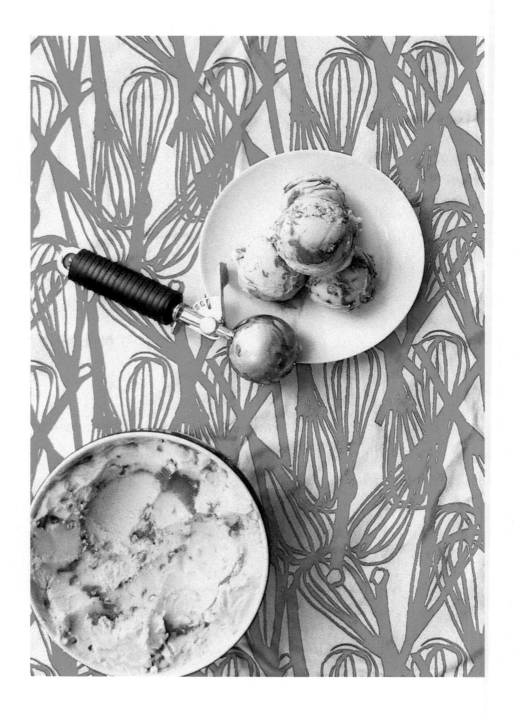

Quick flatbreads with avocado and feta

Ingredients

- 2 ripe avocados
- 250g of whole meal self-rising flour
- 1 teaspoon of rose harissa
- ¾ teaspoon of baking powder
- 75g of feta cheese
- 1 teaspoon cumin seeds
- 350g of plain yoghurt
- Olive oil

Directions

1. Begin by toasting the cumin lightly in a dry pan, place in a bowl.
2. Add the flour together with the baking powder, and yogurt.
3. Season, and mix until dough forms.
4. Turn out onto a lightly floured surface and knead until the dough together.
5. Place in a lightly greased bowl, cover with a damp tea towel, let raise.

6. Chop the avocado into chunks, then place in a bowl.

7. Crumble in the feta with a drizzle of oil, season to taste.

8. In another bowl, stir the harissa into the rest of the yoghurt.

9. Divide the dough into eight balls.

10. Roll each one on a lightly floured surface into an oval shape.

11. Place a griddle pan over a high heat.

12. Griddle each flatbread for 3 minutes, until puffed up.

13. Brush the flatbread with a little oil.

14. Serve and enjoy with the avocado salad and harissa yoghurt.

Smashed avocado, basil, and chicken

Ingredients

- 50g of leftover cooked chicken
- ½ of a ripe avocado
- Extra virgin olive oil
- 2 sprigs of fresh basil

Directions

- Place the avocado in a bowl and mash.
- Pick and tear in the basil leaves.
- Shred the chicken into small pieces.
- Add to the bowl.
- Then, Mix together, and add a little oil to loosen.
- Serve and enjoy.

Cracking cob salad

Ingredients

- 1 large pinch of sweet smoked paprika
- 2 tablespoons of Greek yoghurt
- Olive oil
- 4 slices of pancetta
- 2 large free-range eggs
- 2 free-range chicken thighs
- Extra virgin olive oil
- 1 Romaine, cos lettuce
- ½ teaspoon of Worcestershire sauce
- 1 ripe avocado
- 50ml of buttermilk
- 1 lemon
- 2 ripe tomatoes
- 1 punnet of salad cress
- 50g of Stilton
- ½ a bunch of fresh chives

Directions

1. Preheat the oven to 350°F.
2. Place the chicken thighs into a small roasting tray.

3. Sprinkle over the paprika, and a pinch of sea salt and black pepper.

4. Drizzle over a little olive oil and toss to coat.

5. Let roast for 40 minutes, or until golden, laying over the pancetta for the final 10 minutes. Let cool slightly.

6. Lower the eggs into a pan of vigorously simmering water and boil for 6 minutes, refreshing under cold water, peel.

7. Crumble the Stilton into a large jug.

8. Add chopped chives, with a drizzle of extra virgin olive oil.

9. Squeeze in the lemon juice with the remaining dressing ingredients, whisk.

10. Season to taste with salt and pepper, refrigerate until needed.

11. Remove and discard any tatty outer leaves from the lettuce, chop the rest.

12. Chop avocado, tomatoes, peeled eggs on a board and mix it together.

13. Shred the chicken meat, without bones and skin.

14. Add to the salad.

15. Crumble over the crispy pancetta and continue chopping and mixing together.

16. Transfer the salad to a platter, drizzle over the blue cheese dressing.

17. Serve and enjoy.

Avocado and peas with mashed potato

Ingredients

- 1 sprig of fresh mint
- 1 potato
- 1 large ripe avocado
- 1 tablespoon of milk
- 100g of frozen peas

Directions

1. Peel and dice the potato.
2. Cook in boiling water for 10 minutes.
3. Drain any excess water and mash with the milk.
4. Cook the peas in boiling water for 3 minutes.
5. Drain excess water, place into a bowl, let cool.
6. Add chopped avocado to the bowl.
7. Add the mint leaves and mash together.
8. Serve and enjoy.

Avocado, pancetta, and pine nut salad

Ingredients

- 6 ripe avocados
- Sea salt
- 12 slices pancetta
- 50g of pine nuts
- Balsamic vinegar
- Freshly ground black pepper
- 4 big handfuls of baby spinach
- Extra virgin olive oil

Directions

1. Heat a frying pan and fry the pancetta slices till crispy.
2. Remove from the pan and set aside.
3. In the same pan, lightly toast the pine nuts.
4. Combining balsamic vinegar with olive oil.
5. Season with salt and pepper.
6. Lay out the avocado on a serving plate.
7. Sprinkle over the spinach leaves, pancetta, and toasted pine nuts.

8. Season with salt and pepper and drizzle over your dressing.
9. Serve and enjoy with warm crusty bread.

Roast carrot and avocado salad with orange and lemon dressing

Ingredients

- 2 handfuls of mixed winter salad leaves
- 500g of medium differently colored carrots
- 2 punnet cress
- 1 lemon
- 2 level teaspoons of whole cumin seeds
- 150ml of fat-free natural yoghurt
- 2 small dried chilies
- 3 ripe avocados
- 4 tablespoons of mixed seeds
- 2 cloves garlic
- Red wine vinegar
- 4 sprigs fresh thyme
- 4 x 1cm of thick slices ciabatta
- Extra virgin olive oil
- red or white wine vinegar
- 1 orange

Directions

1. Preheat the oven to 350°F.

2. Boil the carrots in boiling, salted water for 10 minutes.
3. Drain, place into a roasting tray.
4. Mash up the cumin seeds, chilies, salt and pepper in a mortar.
5. Add the garlic with thyme leaves, smash up again until paste foams.
6. Add enough extra virgin olive oil with vinegar to cover the past.
7. Stir together, then pour over the carrots in the tray, to coat.
8. Add the orange and lemon halves, cut-side down.
9. Place in the preheated oven for 30 minutes.
10. Remove the carrots, then add to the avocados.
11. Squeeze the roasted orange and lemon juice into a bowl and add the same amount of extra virgin olive oil, with a swig of red wine vinegar.
12. Season, and pour this dressing over the carrots and avocados.
13. Mix together, taste and adjust the seasoning.
14. Tear the toasted bread into little pieces and add to the dressed carrot and avocado.
15. Serve and enjoy.

Smoked salmon and avocado salad

Ingredients

- Freshly ground black pepper
- 2 small avocados
- 1 lemon
- 200g of smoked salmon
- Sea salt
- ½ cucumber
- 2 handfuls of mixed fresh herbs
- 1 punnet cress
- 2 tablespoons of mixed seeds
- 1 loaf ciabatta
- 1 blood orange
- Extra virgin olive oil

Directions

1. Heat a griddle pan until screaming hot.
2. Place the sliced avocado in a bowl, squeeze over some lemon juice.
3. Slice the cucumber into long, thin strips on top of the avocado.

4. Then, add the herbs and cress.
5. Lightly toast the seeds in a dry pan on a medium to low heat.
6. Squeeze a tablespoon of juice out of the blood orange into a bowl.
7. Add 3 tablespoons of extra virgin olive oil.
8. Season. Mix.
9. Place the ciabatta squares in the griddle pan, charring both sides.
10. Once toasted, drizzle with a little of the dressing and put to one side.
11. Place a square of ciabatta on each of four plates, then top each with a quarter of the smoked salmon.
12. Drizzle the dressing over the salad and mix with your fingertips.
13. Top the smoked salmon with the salad.
14. Serve and enjoy.

Chicken and Soup Mediterranean Sea diet recipes

Chicken among Mediterranean Sea diet foods is at least loved by a huge population; but do you really know how to make it at home without necessarily having to visiting your favorite Mediterranean diet restaurant? There are detailed step-by-step procedures to guide you in making the most tasteful Mediterranean Sea diet chicken recipes.

More so, this book also includes all the fantastic spices to elevate the taste and sweetness of these chicken recipes.

However, all the spices and ingredients you can use in here are natural plants mainly garlic, ginger, cinnamon, lemon, onions, and many others.

Therefore, the following are the chicken and soup Mediterranean Sea diet recipes.

Grilled chicken with charred pineapple salad

Ingredients

- ¼ of a pineapple
- ½ of an avocado
- 1 teaspoon of dried oregano
- ½ a bunch of fresh coriander
- Olive oil
- 1 fresh red chili
- 2 x 150g of free-range chicken breasts
- 2 tablespoons of pickled jalapeños
- 150 g quinoa
- 50g of white cabbage
- 2 limes
- 1 large handful of salad leaves
- 50g of natural yoghurt

Directions

1. Begin by combining the oregano with olive oil in a bowl.
2. Season with sea salt and black pepper.
3. Place the chicken breast with olive oil in the bowl, turning until coated, then leave to one side.

4. Then, cook the quinoa as per the packet Directions, drain, set aside.
5. Place avocado flesh, coriander, jalapeno, and a splash of the pickling liquid and the juice of 1½ limes in a blender.
6. Blend until smooth, stir through the quinoa.
7. Place a griddle pan over a high heat.
8. Place chopped apple on the hot griddle pan for a few minutes on each side.
9. Transfer to a chopping board.
10. In the same pan, griddle the chicken for 5 minutes on each side.
11. Place on the chopping board, let rest and cool.
12. Chop the griddled pineapple into bite-sized chunks, and the chili, then slice the chicken into thin strips.
13. Divide the yoghurt among 4 plates topping with the chicken, and pineapple on one side and the dressed quinoa on the other.
14. Toss the leaves and cabbage with the juice of the remaining lime, chopped chili and a little salt and pepper.
15. Serve and enjoy.

Salina chicken

Ingredients

- 4 sprigs of fresh basil
- 2 red onions
- 3 aubergines
- 1 x 1.4 kg whole free-range chicken
- olive oil
- 200g of ripe cherry tomatoes
- 2 cloves of garlic
- 3 small fresh red chilies
- 50g of pine nuts
- 2 lemons
- 1 cinnamon stick
- 4 sprigs of fresh woody herbs
- 50g of baby capers in brine

Directions

1. Preheat the oven to 350°F.
2. Place chopped aubergines in a large bowl.
3. Then, season with sea salt.
4. Drizzle the chicken pieces with olive oil, place in a large shallow pan on a medium-high heat, with skin side down turning to get golden.

5. Wipe off the salt on aubergines and add to the pan, turning until lightly golden.

6. Remove.

7. Combine garlic with chilies, cinnamon, capers, and woody herbs add to the pan.

8. Stir and fry for briefly, stir in onion, let cook for 15 minutes, stirring occasionally.

9. Squeeze the tomatoes in a bowl of water, remove the seeds.

10. Put the chicken and aubergines back in, drizzle over any resting juices, with half liter of water.

11. Sprinkle over the pine nuts, then squeeze over the lemon juice.

12. Cook at the bottom of the oven until golden.

13. Pick over the basil leaves.

14. Serve and enjoy with lemony couscous.

Chicken tikka skewers

Ingredients

- 3 fresh red chilies
- 2 lemons
- ½ a bunch of fresh coriander
- 2 teaspoons of tikka masala spice paste
- 2 tablespoons of natural yoghurt
- 2 little gem lettuces
- Olive oil
- ½ of a small ripe pineapple
- 2 skinless free-range chicken breasts

Directions

1. Combine lemon juice, olive oil, paste, and yogurt, then mix well.
2. Add sliced pineapple, chilies, sliced chicken to the bowl with the marinade.
3. Toss together to coat, place in the fridge to marinate overnight.
4. Remove the chicken and pineapple mixture from the fridge.
5. Remove and tear the chili into smaller pieces.

6. Starting with the chicken, thread the ingredients onto skewers, alternating between the ingredients.
7. Pour any remaining marinade over the top and drizzle with a little oil.
8. Put a dry pan on a medium heat, then add the skewers, let cook for 10 minutes, turning occasionally, season with a little sea salt.
9. Roughly shave the chicken, pineapple and chili from the skewers with a knife, scatter over the reserved lemon zest and pick over the coriander leaves.
10. Slice the remaining lemon into wedges for squeezing over.
11. Serve and enjoy with the lettuce and yoghurt.

Sticky hoisin chicken

Ingredients

- 3 regular oranges
- 2 x 200g of free-range chicken legs
- 2 heaped tablespoons of hoisin sauce
- 2 fresh mixed-color chilies
- 8 spring onions

Directions

1. Preheat the oven ready to 350°F.
2. Place an ovenproof frying pan on a high heat.
3. Pull off the chicken skin, put both skin and legs into the pan.
4. Season with sea salt and black pepper, letting the fat render out and the chicken get golden, turning halfway.
5. Toss the white spring onions into the pan, after which transfer to the oven for 15 minutes.
6. Place chilies and green spring onions into a bowl of ice-cold water to curl.
7. Arrange sliced oranges on a plates.
8. Remove the chicken skin and soft spring onions from the pan. Set aside.
9. Cook the chicken until tender and cooked through.

10. In a bowl, loosen the hoisin with a splash of red wine vinegar, spoon over the chicken.
11. Sit the chicken and soft spring onions on top and crack over the crispy skin.
12. Serve and enjoy.

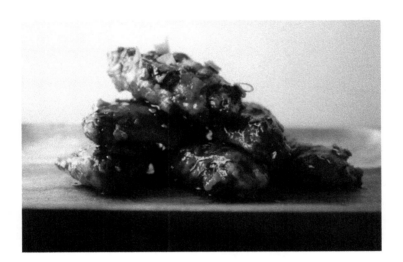

Sweet chicken surprise

Ingredients

- 4 sprigs of fresh tarragon
- 2 x 200g of free-range chicken legs
- 100ml of red vermouth
- 1 bulb of garlic
- 250g of mixed-color seedless grapes

Directions

1. Start by preheating the oven to 350°F.
2. Then, place an ovenproof frying pan over high heat.
3. Rub the chicken with ½ a tablespoon of olive oil.
4. Then, season with sea salt and black pepper and place skin side down in the pan.
5. Fry for a couple of minutes until golden.
6. Squash the unpeeled garlic cloves, add with grapes to the pan.
7. Turn the chicken skin side up, then pour in the vermouth.
8. Transfer to the oven, let roast for 40 minutes, or until the chicken tender.
9. Add a splash of water to the pan and to pick up all the sticky bits.
10. Serve and enjoy.

Sesame butterflied chicken

Ingredients

- 2 tablespoons of natural yoghurt
- 1 tablespoon of low-salt soy sauce
- 100g of fine rice noodles
- 2cm piece of ginger
- 2 x 120g of skinless free-range chicken breasts
- 1 tablespoon of peanut butter
- 2 teaspoons of sesame seeds
- 2 limes
- Groundnut oil
- 4 spring onions
- ½ of a Chinese cabbage
- 200g of sugar snap peas
- 1 fresh red chili

Directions

1. Place your griddle pan over high heat.
2. Then, in a bowl, cover the noodles with boiling kettle water.
3. Rub with 1 teaspoon of groundnut oil on chicken opened up.
4. Season with a small pinch of sea salt and black pepper.

5. Let griddle for 8 minutes, turning halfway.

6. Trim the spring onions and rattle them through the finest slicer on your food processor with the Chinese cabbage, sugar snap peas and chili.

7. Dress with the juice of 1 lime and the soy sauce.

8. In a separate small bowl, mix the peanut butter together with the yoghurt and the juice of the remaining lime, ginger, mix.

9. Slice the chicken on a board, toast lightly with the sesame seeds in the residual heat of the griddle pan.

10. Sprinkle over the chicken.

11. Drain the noodles, divide between plates with the chicken, slaw and peanut sauce, mix.

12. Serve and enjoy.

Chicken and spring green bun cha

Ingredients

- ½ a bunch of fresh mint
- 2 spring onions
- 100g frozen edamame beans
- 1 stick of lemongrass
- 3 tablespoons of vegetable oil
- 5cm piece of ginger
- 1 large fresh red chili
- 200g of baby spinach
- 1½ tablespoons of sesame oil
- 1 tablespoon of low-salt soy sauce
- 150g of broad beans
- 2 tablespoons of runny honey
- 2 tablespoons of hoisin sauce
- 2 limes
- 4 free-range skinless chicken thighs
- 1 tablespoon of rice wine vinegar
- 1 x 225g packet of vermicelli
- 2 large shallots
- ½ a bunch of fresh Thai basil

Directions

1. Preheat the oven to 400°F.
2. Place the lemongrass in a large bowl together with the sesame oil, soy sauce, the zest from 1 lime, honey, hoisin sauce, and the juice from 2 limes. Mix, pour half into a small bowl.
3. Add the chicken to the large bowl, stir and let marinate.
4. Add the rice wine vinegar to the small bowl.
5. Cook defrosted beans in a pan of boiling water for 2 minutes.
6. Drain and rinse under cold water. Set aside.
7. Cook the vermicelli according to the packet Directions, drain.
8. Place the chicken in a small roasting tin lined with tinfoil, move it in the oven heated for 30 minutes.
9. Then, heat olive oil in a small, pan over a medium-high heat.
10. When hot enough, add the shallots, let cook for 5 minutes.
11. Remove, set aside on a tray lined with kitchen paper.
12. Combine the noodles together with the remaining dressing, spring onion, broad beans, baby spinach, and herbs.
13. Top with the chicken, garnished with the shallots.
14. Serve and enjoy.

Firecracker chicken noodle salad

Ingredients

- 1 tablespoon of sweet chili sauce
- 1 tablespoon of coriander oil
- 50g of rice noodles
- ½ tablespoon of low-salt soy sauce
- 1 lime
- 100g of cooked free-range chicken
- ¼ of a cucumber
- 1 carrot
- ½ tablespoon of runny honey
- 1 baby gem lettuce
- 1 small handful of sugar snaps
- A few sprigs of fresh mint
- 1 pinch of mixed seeds

Directions

1. Cook the noodles as instructed on the package.
2. Combine the shredded chicken with the cooked noodles and coriander oil in a bowl.
3. Add all the remaining salad ingredients, toss to combine.
4. Place the sweet chili sauce together with the soy and honey in a small jar. Chill in the lunchbox.

5. Squeeze in the lime juice, secure the lid, keep in the lunchbox.
6. Shake the jam jar to mix the ingredients then dress the salad.
7. Close your lunchbox, shake to coat.
8. Serve and enjoy chilled or at room temperature.

Seared turmeric chicken

Ingredients

- Olive oil
- 200g of seasonal greens
- 2 x 120g of skinless chicken breasts
- 150g of whole wheat couscous
- 2 tablespoons of natural yoghurt
- 2 sprigs of fresh oregano
- ½ a bunch of fresh mint
- 1 lemon
- 1 tablespoon of blanched hazelnuts
- 2 large roasted peeled red peppers in brine
- Hot chili sauce
- 1 level teaspoon of ground turmeric

Directions

1. Combine the oregano leaves, turmeric, olive oil, pinch of salt and black pepper to make a marinade.
2. Then, toss the chicken in the marinade and leave aside.
3. In a boiling water, blanch the greens until tender enough to eat, drain, reserving the water.
4. In a bowl, cover the couscous with boiling greens water, season with a plate on top for 10 minutes.

41

5. Stir chopped mint leaves into the fluffy couscous with the juice of half a lemon.
6. Toast the hazelnuts in a large dry frying pan on a medium-high heat.
7. Remove, and crush in mortar once lightly golden.
8. Return the frying pan to a high heat, let the chicken cook for 4 minutes on each side, turning halfway.
9. Serve the chicken with the couscous, peppers, greens and yoghurt, scattered with the hazelnuts, with a lemon wedge on the side.
10. Enjoy.

Chicken and garlic bread kebabs

Ingredients

- 1 lemon
- 2 sprigs of fresh rosemary
- 2 blood oranges
- 1 tablespoon of balsamic vinegar
- 2 cloves of garlic
- Extra virgin olive oil
- 1 tablespoon white wine vinegar
- 20g of feta cheese
- 8 fresh bay leaves
- Cayenne pepper
- 2 x 120g skinless chicken breasts
- 2 thick slices of whole meal bread
- 100g of baby spinach

Directions

1. Mash up rosemary with a pinch of sea salt in a pestle and mortar. Peel and crush in the garlic, then muddle in 1 tablespoon of oil, the vinegar and a generous pinch of cayenne.
2. Place chopped chicken and bread in a bowl, toss to mix well with the marinade until evenly coated.

3. Place the frying pan on a medium-high heat.

4. Then, lay the skewers in the pan, let cook for 5 minutes on each side.

5. Dress the spinach with a squeeze of lemon juice and a drizzle of olive oil.

6. Organize on the plates with the blood oranges and drizzle with the balsamic.

7. Serve and enjoy topped with the kebabs and lemon wedges.

Piri piri chicken

Ingredients

- 1.3kg of chicken
- 3 sprigs of fresh thyme
- 4 cloves of garlic
- Olive oil
- 2 red onions
- 4 ripe mixed-color tomatoes
- 6 fresh mixed-color chilies
- Red wine vinegar
- Extra virgin olive oil
- 750g of sweet potatoes
- 2 teaspoons of smoked paprika
- 2 tablespoons of fine semolina
- 1 x 200g jar of pickled jalapeños
- 1 bunch of fresh coriander

Directions

1. Combine thyme leaves, garlic, paprika, and a pinch of sea salt in a pestle and mortar.
2. Blend to foam paste, add 2 tablespoons of olive oil.
3. Rub the marinade on the chicken.

4. Cover properly, and refrigerate to marinate overnight or more than, two hours, if one has no time.

5. Preheat the oven to 350°F.

6. Then, place a large griddle pan over a high heat.

7. Place unpeeled onions and tomatoes, chilies, and unpeeled garlic on the hot griddle.

8. Let, grill for 10 minutes, turning regularly.

9. Remove the garlic skins and peel the onions.

10. Add every vegetable to a food processor with a splash of red wine vinegar and extra virgin olive oil.

11. Blend until smooth, adjusting with water if too thick.

12. Season, and adjust.

13. Return the griddle pan to a high heat, then add the marinated chicken and sear all over for 10 minutes, turning regularly.

14. Then, transfer to a roasting tray, put in the hot oven for 45 minutes.

15. Toss the sweet potatoes with the paprika, semolina, extra virgin olive oil, a small pinch of salt and black pepper.

16. Spread the wedges out on 2 large baking trays.

17. Place in the oven for 30 minutes, or until tender and crisp.

18. Drain and add the jalapeños to a food processor with a splash of the pickling juice.

19. Tear in the coriander with a splash of extra virgin olive oil.

20. Blend until smooth.

21. Serve the roast chicken with piri piri sauce, sweet potato wedges and a little jalapeño salsa.

22. Enjoy.

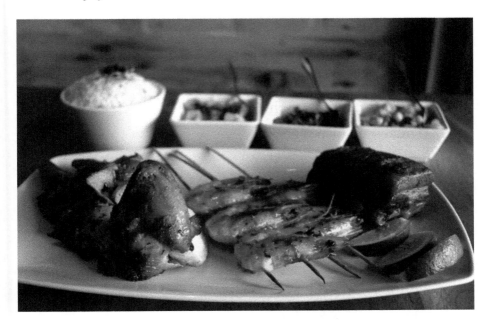

Blackened chicken

Ingredients

- Olive oil
- 1 heaped teaspoon of ground allspice
- 300g of quinoa
- 2 x 200g of skinless chicken breasts
- 2 mixed-color peppers
- 1 fresh red chili
- 4 tablespoons of fat-free yoghurt
- 1 punnet cress
- 100g of baby spinach
- 4 spring onions
- 1 bunch of fresh coriander
- 1 bunch of fresh mint
- 1 large ripe mango
- 2 limes
- 2 tablespoons of extra virgin olive oil
- 1 ripe avocado
- 50g of feta cheese
- 1 heaped teaspoon of smoked paprika

Directions

1. Firstly, put the quinoa into the pan and generously cover with boiling water.
2. Combine the chili together with the spinach, spring onions, leafy mint, and coriander into the processor, blend until finely chopped.
3. Toss the chicken with sea salt, black pepper, the allspice, and paprika on a greaseproof pan.
4. Fold over the paper, then flatten the chicken.
5. Place into the frying pan with 1 tablespoon of olive oil, turning after 4 minutes.
6. Then, add peppers to the frying pan, tossing regularly.
7. Drain the quinoa, place on to a serving board.
8. Toss with the blended spinach mixture, squeeze over the lime juice.
9. Add the extra virgin olive oil, mix and season to taste.
10. Sprinkle the mango chunks and cooked peppers over the quinoa.
11. Scoop curls of avocado flesh over the salad.
12. Slice up the chicken, toss the slices in any juices, then add to the salad.
13. Crumble over the feta, scatter over the remaining coriander leaves.
14. Serve and enjoy with a dollop of yoghurt.

Pukka yellow curry

Ingredients

- Natural yoghurt
- 2 onions
- 1 teaspoon of tomato puree
- 1 level teaspoon of ground turmeric
- 4 cloves of garlic
- 1 lemon
- 2 teaspoons of curry powder
- 5cm piece of ginger
- 2 yellow peppers
- 1 organic chicken stock cube
- Olive oil
- 1 mug of basmati rice
- 2 fresh red chilies
- ½ a bunch of fresh coriander
- 1 teaspoon of runny honey
- 8 chicken drumsticks
- 1 x 400 g tin of chickpeas

Directions

1. Place 1 onion, pepper, garlic, and ginger into a food processor.

2. Then, crumble in the stock cube with the chili, coriander stalks, honey, and spices. Blend until paste forms.
3. Place a large casserole pan on a medium-high heat.
4. Fry the chicken drumsticks with a splash of olive oil for 10 minutes, turning occasionally.
5. Remove the chicken to a plate, leaving the pan on the heat.
6. Add the remaining onion and pepper to the pan, let cook briefly.
7. Then place in the paste, let cook for 5 minutes.
8. Pour in 500ml of boiling water.
9. Drain the chickpeas, add with the tomato puree and a pinch of sea salt and black pepper, then stir.
10. Return the chicken to the pan, cover, simmer gently for 45 minutes over low heat.
11. Place in 1 mug of rice with 2 mugs of boiling water into a pan with a pinch of salt let simmer for 12 minutes covered.
12. Serve and enjoy.

Roasted chicken breast with lemony Bombay potatoes

Ingredients

- Olive oil
- 200g of potatoes
- A few sprigs of fresh coriander
- 2cm piece of ginger
- ¼ teaspoon of ground turmeric
- ½ red pepper
- 1 free-range chicken breast
- ½ teaspoon of ground cumin
- 1 lemon

Directions

1. Preheat the oven to 400°F.
2. Cook the potatoes in boiling salted water for 6 minutes, drain and steam dry.
3. Add the turmeric, cumin, coriander leaves, ginger, pepper, grate lemon zest to a bowl.
4. Squeeze a little juice from the remainder of the lemon into the bowl.

5. Shake the potatoes up in the colander, add to the bowl with the chicken.
6. Drizzle with olive oil.
7. Season with sea salt and black pepper, toss to coat.
8. Remove the chicken from the bowl, place the potato mixture into a baking dish.
9. Spread out into a single layer topping with the lemon slices, then drape over the chicken.
10. Drizzle with olive oil, cook in the middle of the oven for 25 minutes.
11. Serve and enjoy.

Chicken and squash cacciatore

Ingredients

- 8 black olives
- 250ml of Chianti
- 1 onion
- 4 chicken thighs, bone in
- 1 leek
- 4 cloves of garlic
- 200g of seeded whole meal bread
- Olive oil
- 2 fresh bay leaves
- 2 sprigs of fresh rosemary
- ½ a butternut squash
- 100g of shell nut mushrooms
- 2 rashers of smoked pancetta
- 2 x 400g tins of plum tomatoes

Directions

1. Preheat your oven to 375°F.
2. Place a large ovenproof casserole pan on a medium heat.
3. Place sliced pancetta, rosemary leaves, 1 tablespoon of olive oil, onion, garlic, bay leaves, and leek in the pan. Stir regularly for 10 minutes.

4. Add the stalk with the whole mushrooms, squash to the pan.
5. Remove and discard the chicken skin and add the chicken to the pan.
6. Pour in the wine, let reduce slightly.
7. Add the tomatoes and break them up with a wooden spoon.
8. Half-fill each tin with water, swirl about, pour into the pan, mix.
9. Destone and poke the olives into the stew.
10. Bring to a gentle simmer.
11. Transfer to the oven, let cook for 1 hour.
12. Season, and adjust accordingly.
13. Serve and enjoy.

Barbecued chicken

Ingredients

- 24 ripe cherry tomatoes
- 2 sprigs of fresh rosemary
- Olive oil
- 1 lemon
- 1 teaspoon of wholegrain mustard
- 400g of green beans
- 4 skinless chicken breasts
- Extra virgin olive oil

Directions

1. Preheat the oven to 200°F.
2. Place rosemary leaves and a pinch of sea salt in a mortar, bash well.
3. Add the grated lemon zest and squeeze in half the juice with 2 tablespoons of olive oil.
4. Open the chicken breast and flatten
5. Pour the rosemary marinade over the chicken, let marinate briefly.
6. Mix the mustard with the remaining lemon juice and more extra virgin olive oil.

7. Place the tomatoes onto a tray, season, roast for 20 minutes.
8. Cook the beans in a pan of boiling salted water for 5 minutes.
9. Drain, toss in the mustard dressing, add the roasted tomatoes.
10. Preheat a barbecue.
11. Barbecue the chicken breasts for 5 minutes, turning regularly.
12. Serve and enjoy with beans and tomatoes.

All in one rice and chicken

Ingredients

- 250g of long-grain rice
- Olive oil
- 2 teaspoons of ground coriander
- 1 tablespoon of runny honey
- 2 chicken legs
- A few sprigs of fresh coriander
- 2 chicken thighs
- 1 onion
- 1 clove of garlic
- 1 heaped teaspoon of ground cumin
- 150g of dates

Directions

1. Heat a splash of olive oil, then brown the chicken legs and thighs in a pan. Remove.
2. Add diced onion, let sweet, then add crushed garlic with the spices in the same a pan.
3. Let cook for 2 minutes, stir in the rice together with the dates, honey, and browned chicken.
4. Cover with water, let boil, then let simmer, for 30 minutes covered over low heat.

5. Season with sea salt and black pepper.
6. Scatter over the chopped coriander leaves.
7. Serve and enjoy.

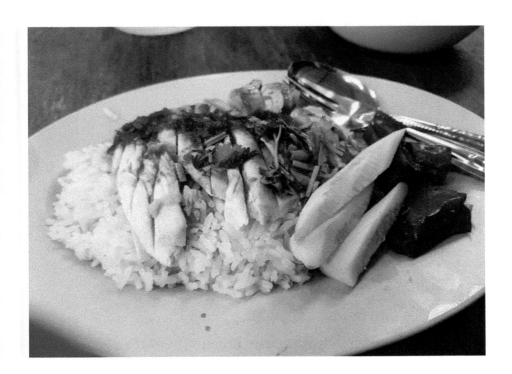

Spinach and tortellini soup

Ingredients

- 1 large handful of spinach
- 200g of tortellini
- 1-liter organic chicken
- 2 fresh bay leaves
- 50g of frozen peas

Directions

1. Firstly, pour the stock into a large pan.
2. Then, add the bay leaves, bring to the boil.
3. Add the tortellini, let cook for 4 minutes.
4. Add the peas, let cook for a further 3 minutes.
5. Add the spinach and cook until wilted.
6. Place into bowls.
7. Serve and enjoy with crusty bread.

Warm potato, herring, beetroot and apple salad

Ingredients

- 4 tablespoons of olive oil
- 200g of beetroot
- 2 tablespoons of red wine vinegar
- 1 pinch of granulated sugar
- 500g of Ratte potatoes
- A few fresh chives
- 1 small apple
- 1 lug of sparkling water
- 2 marinated herring fillets
- ½ tablespoon of Dijon mustard

1. **Directions**
2. For the vinaigrette, combine the Dijon mustard together with the olive oil, red wine vinegar, and sugar in a bowl.
3. Season with sea salt and black pepper, then whisk to blend.
4. Add the sparkling water to loosen the mixture, then whisk.

5. Cook the beetroot in a pan of boiling salted water for 45 minutes.
6. In another separate pan of boiling salted water, cook unpeeled potatoes for 20 minutes. Drain in a colander, then slice warm.
7. Drain and allow the beetroot to cool slightly, then slice.
8. Divide the potato, beetroot, apple slices and herring fillets among 4 serving plates.
9. Drizzle over the vinaigrette, chop and scatter over the chives.
10. Serve and enjoy with warm potatoes.

Beetroot dip

Ingredients

- 4 vac-packed beetroot
- 1 tablespoon of horseradish
- Rye bread
- 1 teaspoon of caraway seeds
- 3 sprigs of fresh thyme
- 3 tablespoons of crème fraiche

Directions

1. Pick the thyme leaves, and blend all the ingredients in a food processor.
2. Season with sea salt and black pepper.
3. Serve and enjoy with rye bread.
4. 374. Beetroot, almond, and ricotta
5. Ingredients
6. 2 tablespoons of ground almonds
7. 2 tablespoons of ricotta cheese
8. Vac-packed cooked beetroot
9. Directions
10. Place the beetroot in a blender.
11. Add the ground almonds together with the ricotta cheese to the blender, a purée.

63

12. Adjust thickness with water.

13. Serve and enjoy.

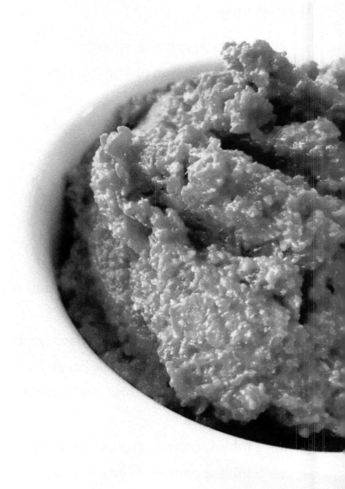

Chili pickled sweet and sour beets

Ingredients

- 3 fresh red chillies
- 100ml of balsamic vinegar
- 1 tablespoon coriander seeds
- 400ml of white wine vinegar
- 200g of golden caster sugar
- 1/2 lemon
- 1.5 kg of beetroots

Directions

1. Place the beets in a pan of salted water and bring to the boil.
2. Let simmer for 30 minutes until cooked, then drain. Let cool.
3. Add the vinegars together with the sugar in a separate pan.
4. Add halved chilies to the pan with a squeeze of lemon juice, coriander seeds, and a pinch of sea salt, over a high heat.
5. Bring to the boil, stirring until the sugar is dissolved.

6. Spoon the beets into jars, pour the pickling liquid on top.
7. Add a chili to each jar, seal, infuse for few days
8. Serve and enjoy.

Beetroot, peach, and coconut no cook recipe

Ingredients

- 100 ml of coconut milk
- 1 whole ripe peach
- 1 vac-packed cooked beetroot

Directions

1. Place peeled peach in a blender.
2. Add the beetroot.
3. Pour in the coconut milk, blend until smooth.
4. Adjust its thickness with water.
5. Serve and enjoy.

Pink risotto

Ingredients

- ½ x 220g tin of chopped tomatoes
- ½ of a small onion
- 50g of basmati rice
- 2 vac-packed beetroot
- ½ tablespoon of olive oil

Directions

1. Heat the olive oil in a medium pan over medium heat.
2. Add the onions, let fry for 5 minutes.
3. Then, add the rice stirring until well coated.
4. Pour in boiling water, cook for 8 minutes covered.
5. Stir in the beetroot together with the tomatoes.
6. Lower the heat, let cook until all the liquid has been absorbed.
7. Then, mash until fairly smooth, with some soft lumps.
8. Serve and enjoy.

Vegan beetroot carpaccio

Ingredients

- 2 tablespoons of olive oil
- 8 medium beetroots
- 2 lemons
- 2 teaspoons of caster sugar
- 1 tablespoon of capers
- ½ a bunch of fresh dill
- 1 red onion

Directions

1. Place the beetroot in a large saucepan, then cover with water.
2. Bring to the boil, lower the heat, let simmer gently, for 40 minutes, covered partially. Drain and set aside.
3. Into a bowl, grate the zest of one of the lemons, then squeeze in the juice from both, passing it through a fine sieve.
4. Add chopped dill, sugar, olive oil, capers, sea salt, and onion to the bowl. Whisk until fully amalgamated.
5. Run the beetroots under a cold tap and gently slide off the skins.
6. Then, slice the beetroot into thin rounds.

7. Arrange the beetroot slices on a serving platter.

8. Spoon over the dressing, allow it to sink into the crevice of the beetroots.

9. Then, cover with Clingfilm, place in the fridge for 4 hours.

10. Remove, serve and enjoy.

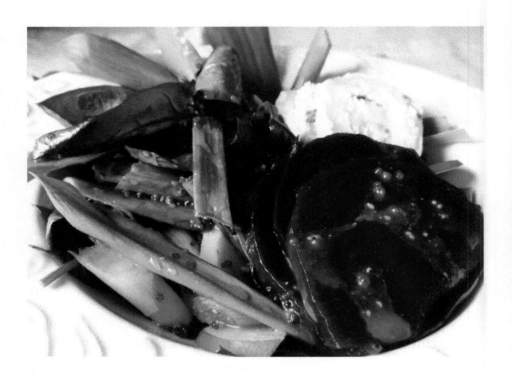

Candied beet salad

Ingredients

- 75ml of buttermilk
- 750g of golden beetroot
- 150g of golden caster sugar
- Juice of 1 lemon
- 50g of mixed seeds
- Extra virgin olive oil
- 1/2 teaspoon of sweet smoked paprika
- 1/2 bunch of mixed soft herbs
- 2 knobs of unsalted butter
- Zest and juice of 1 orange
- 1/4 teaspoon of ground cinnamon
- 2 handfuls of salad leaves

Directions

1. Place the beets in water, bring to the boil over a high heat, reduce heat let simmer and cook for 1 hour.
2. Drain, let cool. then, peel off the skins and roughly cut into 3cm wedges.
3. Toss the seeds in a little olive oil with the paprika and a pinch of sea salt and black pepper.
4. Toast in a dry frying pan until golden.

5. Whisk the buttermilk in a jug together with the juice of half the lemon, and olive oil. Season.

6. Stir into the dressing chopped herbs, place to one side.

7. Melt the butter in the same frying pan used for toasting the seeds.

8. Finely grate in the zest of the orange.

9. Add a squeeze of orange juice together with the cinnamon, sugar, and a pinch of salt and pepper.

10. Bring to the boil and leave to bubble away for 10 minutes.

11. Remove from the heat and toss through the cooked beets.

12. Toss the salad leaves with the buttermilk dressing and scatter over the beets.

13. Serve and enjoy with the toasted seeds.

Rainbow salad wrap

Ingredients

- 3 teaspoons of cider vinegar
- 2 small raw beetroots
- 50g of feta cheese
- 2 carrots
- 5 tablespoons of natural yogurt
- 150g of white cabbage
- 2 tablespoons of extra virgin olive oil
- 1 pear
- ½ a bunch of fresh mint
- ½ teaspoon of English mustard
- ½ a bunch of parsley
- 6 small whole meal tortilla wraps

Directions

1. Firstly, place the grated carrots, cabbage, pear, mint, parsley leaves, and beetroots into a large bowl.
2. Add natural yogurt, English mustard, cider vinegar, and extra virgin olive oil to a jam jar.
3. Secure the lid and shake well.
4. Taste and adjust accordingly.
5. Drizzle most of the dressing over the salad.

6. Divide the salad between the tortilla wraps, crumble a little feta over each.
7. Roll up the wraps, tucking them in at the sides.
8. Serve and enjoy.

Mandolin salad

Ingredients

- ½ Bunch of fresh mint
- 50ml of milk
- 3 large raw beetroots
- Rapeseed oil
- 2 apples
- 200g of soft goat's cheese
- Cider vinegar

Directions

1. Begin by whisking the goat's cheese together with the milk in a food processor until blended with a thick cream.
2. Season with sea salt and black pepper.
3. Spoon over a large platter.
4. Toss sliced beets and apples together with a little drizzle of olive oil and a tiny splash of cider vinegar.
5. Pile it all on top of the goat's cheese mix.
6. Sprinkle sliced mint over.
7. Serve and enjoy immediately.

Gorgeous roast vegetables

Ingredients

- Sea salt
- 800g of mixed-color carrot
- Freshly ground black pepper
- 800g of potatoes
- 350g of parsnips
- 6 tablespoon of duck fat
- 350g of raw beetroot
- A few sprigs of fresh rosemary

Directions

1. Start by dividing the vegetables between a few large pans, cover with boiling salted water and parboil for 15 minutes.
2. Drain in a large colander, steam dry for some minutes.
3. Shake the colander to chuff up the edges, place in the largest roasting tray.
4. Drizzle with the duck fat, put the rosemary leaves over.
5. Season with salt and pepper, toss to coat.
6. Push the vegetables into a single layer.
7. At 425°F, cook for 40 minutes or so, turning halfway through.
8. Serve and enjoy with the roast duck.

Root vegetable salad

Ingredients

- Freshly ground black pepper
- Sea salt
- 3 carrots
- 3 raw beetroots
- 1 fennel bulb
- 5 tablespoons of extra virgin olive oil
- 1 bunch of radishes
- 1 celery heart
- ½ a bunch of fresh mint
- ½ a small radicchio
- 1 lemon

Directions

1. Place the carrots with beetroots, radishes, celery, lettuce, fennel bulbs in a large mixing bowl.
2. Squeeze lemon juice into a small bowl, add mind leaves with extra virgin olive oil.
3. Whisk together with a fork, then shake well.
4. Taste the dressing, adjust the season with a tiny pinch of salt and pepper.
5. Pour over the root vegetables.

6. Toss the vegetables in the dressing.

7. Transfer to a serving bowl and sprinkle over the fennel tops and reserved baby mint.

8. Serve and enjoy.

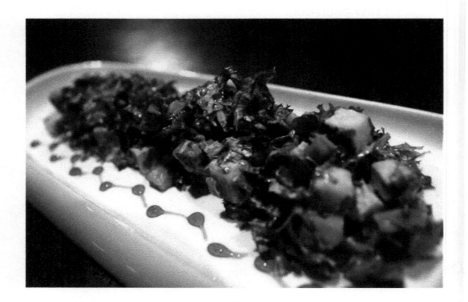

Home-cured beetroot gravadlax

Ingredients

- 1 loaf of brown bread
- 2 large fresh beetroots
- A few handfuls of watercress
- 50ml of gin
- 1 orange
- 2 lemons
- 2 juniper berries
- 1 lemon, cut into wedges
- 6 tablespoons of rock salt
- 1 small bunch fresh tarragon
- 2 tablespoons of demerara sugar
- 50ml of gin
- 800g of side of salmon
- 1 small bunch fresh dill
- 4 tablespoons of freshly grated horseradish

Directions

1. Blend the beetroots together with the orange, lemon zest, and juniper berries in a food processor until fairly smooth paste forms.
2. Transfer this to a bowl and stir in the rock salt and sugar.

3. Pour in the gin and mix.

4. Lay the salmon with the skin-side down on a large baking tray.

5. Gently pour over the beetroot cure.

6. Spread all over the salmon flesh in a uniform manner.

7. Then, wrap the salmon in a double layer of greaseproof paper, wrap with Clingfilm.

8. Refrigerate for 24 hours.

9. Take the salmon out of the fridge, unwrap to rinse off the cure.

10. Push the beetroot cure off the fish.

11. Place the rinsed salmon to one side and run the tray under the tap.

12. Mix together the chopped herbs, horseradish, and gin.

13. Put the salmon back into the clean tray, skin-side down.

14. Pack the herby cure onto the salmon using your hands.

15. Wrap with a double layer of greaseproof paper, refrigerate for 24 hours.

16. The following day your salmon will be perfectly cured and ready to eat.

17. Serve and enjoy.

Roasted vegetable mega mix

Ingredients

- 5 fresh bay leaves
- 2 bulbs of fennel
- Olive oil
- 350g of beetroot
- A few sprigs of fresh thyme
- 2 balsamic vinegar
- A few sprigs of fresh oregano
- White wine vinegar
- 500g of carrots
- 1 clementine
- A few sprigs of fresh rosemary
- 400g of parsnips
- ½ of a lemon
- 3 sprigs of fresh sage
- 1 small teaspoon of runny honey
- 350g of baby turnips
- 2 of red wine vinegar

Directions

1. Preheat your oven to 375°F.
2. Bring two large pans of salted water to the boil.

3. Place beets in one of the pans, keep separated from the rest of the vegetables. Boil for 25 minutes or so.
4. Place carrots, parsnips, and fennel in the second pan, boil for 10 minutes.
5. Drain, let steam dry, then separate to hit them with those different flavors.
6. Toss the beets with the balsamic vinegar and whole herb sprigs.
7. Toss the carrots with the clementine juice, place in the squeezed halves, pick over the rosemary leaves.
8. Toss the parsnips with the vinegar and tear over the sage leaves.
9. Toss the turnips with the vinegar and bay.
10. Toss the fennel with the lemon juice, place over the thyme leaves.
11. Lay them out on a large tray, according to veggie types.
12. Let roast until golden and crispy.
13. Drizzle with the honey over the parsnips the veggies are about to get ready.
14. Serve and enjoy.

Rainbow trout with horseradish yogurt and balsamic beets

Ingredients

- 4 jarred beetroots
- 400g of potatoes
- 1 heaped teaspoon of creamed horseradish
- Balsamic vinegar
- Sea salt
- 2 handfuls of watercress
- Freshly ground black pepper
- 4 x 100g of rainbow trout fillets
- Extra virgin olive oil
- 2 heaped tablespoons of natural yoghurt
- Olive oil
- A few sprigs fresh thyme
- 1 lemon

Directions

1. Add the potatoes to a pan of salted boiling water, let cook for 15 minutes.
2. Put a large frying pan on a medium heat.

3. Then, season the trout on both sides with a pinch of salt and pepper.
4. Add olive oil to the pan, scatter in the thyme tips, trout.
5. Press down on the fish to crisp up the skin, let cook for 4 minutes.
6. In a small bowl, mix the yoghurt together with the juice of ½ a lemon, horseradish, and a small pinch of salt.
7. Dress the beets with a splash of balsamic and a small pinch of salt.
8. Drain the potatoes, toss with a pinch of salt and pepper and a drizzle of olive oil.
9. Serve and enjoy with a dollop of yogurt, radish, and drizzle of extra virgin olive oil.

Raw beetroot salad

Ingredients

- Fresh horseradish
- Pepper
- Beetroots
- Salt
- Flat-leaf parsley

Directions

1. Combine sliced beets with flavors, chopped parsley leaves, salt, pepper, and grated horseradish.
2. Let rest for 10 minutes to allow the horseradish to soften the beetroot.
3. Toss with a splash of vodka.
4. Serve and enjoy.

Fresh smoked salmon and beetroot salad

Ingredients

- Balsamic vinegar
- 4 raw baby beetroot
- 2cm piece of fresh horseradish
- ½ lemon
- Sea salt
- Freshly ground black pepper
- 1 loaf of granary bread
- Extra virgin olive oil
- 200g of smoked salmon
- 35g of watercress

Directions

1. Begin by shaving the beetroot into a bowl.
2. Then, add the lemon juice with a small pinch of salt and pepper, extra virgin olive oil, and a splash of balsamic vinegar, mix well
3. Organize the smoked salmon in waves over a large platter.

4. Then, Scatter over the watercress, then the beetroot slices, leaving any juices behind in the bowl.
5. Over the beetroot, grate the horseradish, then spoon the juices from the beetroot over the top.
6. Sprinkle with an extra pinch of pepper and a drizzle of extra virgin olive oil.
7. Serve and enjoy with fresh loaf of granary bread.

Crunchy raw beetroot salad with feta and pear

Ingredients

- 1 lemon
- 3 ripe pears
- Extra virgin olive oil
- 4 large beetroot
- A few sprigs of fresh mint
- 1 large handful of sunflower seeds
- 200g of feta cheese

Directions

1. Squeeze the lemon juice into a clean jam jar.
2. Top with 10 tablespoons of oil, and a pinch of sea salt and black pepper.
3. Shake the jar once the lid is secured, keep aside until needed.
4. Dress the matchsticks in a little of the lemon oil dressing.
5. Taste, and adjust the flavors and seasoning.
6. Divide the salad between plates, crumble over the creamy feta.

7. Sprinkle chopped mint leaves over the salad with the sunflower seeds.

8. Serve and enjoy.

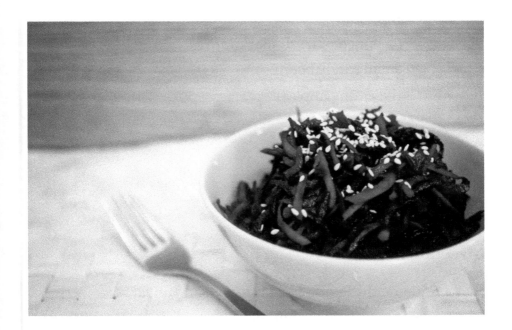

Beetroot, red apple, and watercress salad

Ingredients

- 1 small handful of pea shoots
- 2 small red beetroot
- ½ a bunch of fresh marjoram
- 2 small candy beetroot
- 2 red eating apples
- ½ of a lemon
- extra virgin olive oil
- 1 bag of rocket
- 40g of watercress

Directions

1. Squeeze the lemon juice into a clean jam jar.
2. Add three times the amount of extra virgin olive oil.
3. Then, season with sea salt and black pepper.
4. Fasten or secure the lid and shake to emulsify.
5. Add the rocket together with the watercress, pea shoots, beetroot, and apples to a large bowl.
6. Drizzle over enough dressing to coat the ingredients.
7. Place in the marjoram leaves, toss again.
8. Serve and enjoy.

Avocado pastry quiche

Ingredients

- 2 ripe avocados
- 100g bag of mixed salad
- Extra virgin olive oil
- 400g of self-raising flour
- 1 lemon
- Olive oil
- 6 large free-range eggs
- 300g of frozen peas
- 90g of cheddar cheese
- ½ a bunch of basil

Directions

1. Preheat the oven to 400°F
2. In a large bowl, smash up the avocado, then rub in the flour with a pinch of sea salt and 4 tablespoons of cold water until it foams a dough.
3. Knead until smooth.
4. Wrap and rest for 15 minutes.
5. Crack the eggs into a blender, add the frozen peas and most of the Cheddar.

6. Place basil leaves with a pinch of salt and black pepper, blend until smooth.
7. Roll out the avocado pastry on a flour-dusted surface.
8. Loosely roll it up around the rolling pin, then unroll it over an oiled baking tray.
9. Let bake for 10 minutes, or until lightly golden.
10. Pour in the filling and bake for another 15 minutes.
11. Dress the salad leaves with extra virgin olive oil and lemon juice.
12. Season, and sprinkle over the quiche.
13. Serve and enjoy.

Fluffy flourless pancake

Ingredients

- 2 large free-range eggs
- Chili sauce
- 2 large free-range eggs
- 100g of porridge oats
- 1 teaspoon of baking powder
- Olive oil
- 100g of cottage cheese
- 1 avocado

Directions

1. Put the oats together with the cottage cheese, 2 eggs, and the baking powder in a blender, process until smooth with a tiny pinch of sea salt.
2. Heat a large non-stick frying pan over a medium-high heat with a small splash of oil.
3. Add the batter to the pan, little by little at a time.
4. Let fry for 2 minutes, or until golden, flipping halfway.
5. Serve and enjoy topping with sliced avocado, a fried egg and chili sauce.

Roasted black beans burgers

This incredible fruity recipe features mangos and tabasco with beans and zingy tomato perfect for a Mediterranean Sea diet.

Ingredients

- 1 ripe avocado
- 200g of mixed mushrooms
- 4 tablespoons of natural yoghurt
- 100g of rye bread
- Chipotle tabasco sauce
- Ground coriander
- 1 x 400g tin of black beans
- 4 sprigs of fresh coriander
- 1 lime
- Olive oil
- 40g of mature cheddar cheese
- 1 ripe mango
- 1½ red onions
- 4 soft rolls
- 100g of ripe cherry tomatoes

Directions

1. First, preheat the oven ready to 400°F.
2. Combine onion, rye bread, mushroom, and 1 teaspoon of coriander in a food processor, blend until fine.
3. Drain and pulse in the black beans.
4. Then, season lightly with sea salt and black pepper.
5. Divide into 4 and shape into patties.
6. Rub all over with oil and dust with ground coriander.
7. Transfer to an oiled baking tray, let roast for 25 minutes, or until dark.
8. Place remaining chopped onion, tomato in a bowl.
9. Then, squeeze over the lime juice, with few shakes of Tabasco and season to taste.
10. Halve the warm rolls and divide the yoghurt between the bases, with salsa, mango, avocado, and coriander leaves.
11. Top with the burgers, remaining salsa and extra Tabasco.
12. Serve and enjoy.

Mexican baked eggs

Ingredients

- ½ a lime
- 4 large free-range eggs
- 1 red chili
- Olive oil
- 2 sprigs of fresh coriander
- 1 ripe avocado

Directions

1. Preheat the oven to high hot.
2. Then, grease a small skillet pan with a drizzle of olive oil, crack in the eggs.
3. Scatter sliced red chili over the eggs.
4. juice of one half.
5. Organize the avocado around the eggs.
6. Season with a little sea salt and black pepper.
7. Place in the oven for 10 minutes, or until the egg whites are set.
8. Sprinkle some coriander leaves over the eggs.
9. Cut the remaining lime into wedges, squeeze over.
10. Serve and enjoy with hot buttered toast.

Crispy squid and smashed avocado

Ingredients

- 2 limes
- 2 heaped tablespoons of whole meal flour
- 1 ripe avocado
- 2 teaspoons of hot chili sauce
- 250g of squid, gutted, cleaned

Directions

1. Pour olive oil into a large frying pan on a medium-high heat, let heat up.
2. Toss all the squid with the flour and a pinch of sea salt and black pepper to coat.
3. Scoop the avocado flesh into a bowl.
4. Grate in the zest of 1 lime, squeeze in the juice and mash until smooth.
5. Taste, an adjust the seasoning.
6. Piece by piece, place the remaining squid in the hot oil, cook until golden all over.
7. Remove to a plate lined with kitchen paper to drain excess olive oil.
8. Drizzle over the chili sauce and a little extra virgin olive oil.

9. Serve and enjoy with lime wedges.

Avocado on rye toast with ricotta

Ingredients

- 1 teaspoon of toasted pine nuts
- 1 ripe tomato
- 1 heaped teaspoon of ricotta cheese
- 1 lemon
- 1 sprig of fresh basil
- 1 x 75g slice of rye bread
- ½ of a ripe avocado

Directions

1. Begin by spreading the ricotta cheese over the rye bread.
2. Then, slice the avocado with tomato,
3. Toss with a squeeze of lemon juice.
4. Season accordingly and arrange on the toast.
5. Sprinkle over the pine nuts and a few fresh baby basil leaves.
6. Serve and enjoy.

Avocado on rye toast with chocolate

Ingredients

- Raspberries
- ½ of a ripe avocado
- Dark chocolate
- ½ of a ripe banana
- 1 x 75g slice of rye bread
- 1 heaped teaspoon of light cream cheese
- 2 teaspoons of toasted hazelnuts
- 1 teaspoon of cocoa powder

Directions

1. Smash up the avocado together with the banana, cream cheese, and cocoa powder until smooth.
2. Spread over the rye bread.
3. Dot over a few raspberries with the toasted hazelnuts.
4. Shave over a tiny bit of dark chocolate.
5. Serve and enjoy.

Mega veggie nachos

This is a favorite for most vegetarians and other Mediterranean Sea diet lovers.

It features variety of fruits and vegetables along with herbs for a perfect taste and flavor.

Ingredients

- 1 ripe avocado
- 1 fresh red chili
- 1 x 400g tin of black beans
- 3 ripe tomatoes
- 20g of feta cheese
- 6 spring onions
- 1 bunch of fresh coriander
- 2 limes
- 2 mixed-color peppers
- Chipotle Tabasco sauce
- Extra virgin olive oil
- 4 corn tortillas
- ½ teaspoon of cumin seeds

Directions

1. Place the oven on to 350°F.

2. Place a griddle pan over a high heat and cook the whole peppers, together with chili, tomatoes, and trimmed spring onions until charred.

3. Place the peppers and chili in a bowl, cover with Clingfilm, set aside briefly.

4. Combine tomatoes, spring onions, peppers, and chilies in a bowl.

5. Season few coriander leaves, then mix in a squeeze of lime juice and a drizzle of oil.

6. Cut the tortillas into wedges and arrange over the baking sheets.

7. Let bake for 5 minutes and or until golden.

8. Toast the cumin seeds over high heat.

9. Add the Tabasco sauce with beans, cook for a few minutes, stirring occasionally.

10. Drizzle avocado wedges with the remaining lime juice.

11. Arrange the tortillas in a bowl.

12. Top with the beans, salsa, dressed avocado, feta.

13. Serve and enjoy.

Avocado on rye toast with beetroot

Ingredients

- ½ of a ripe avocado
- 1 beetroot
- 1 teaspoon of extra virgin olive oil
- 1 teaspoon of mixed seeds
- 1 teaspoon of hummus
- 1 teaspoon of cottage cheese
- 1 x 75g of slice of rye bread

Directions

1. Start by smashing up the beetroot together with the hummus and cottage cheese.
2. Season to taste and spread over the rye bread.
3. Place ripe avocado on top.
4. Drizzle with the extra virgin olive oil.
5. Sprinkle with mixed seeds.
6. Serve and enjoy.

Baked sweet potatoes, avocado, and queso fresco

Ingredients

- 150g of Mexican queso fresco
- 4 sweet potatoes
- 2 limes
- Olive oil
- 1 handful of pumpkin seeds
- 2 ripe avocados

Directions

1. Preheat the oven ready to 380°F.
2. Drizzle the potatoes with oil.
3. Season with a sprinkle of sea salt and black pepper.
4. Wrap in a foil and bake in the oven for 1 hour and 15 minutes.
5. When the potatoes are nearly done, destone and roughly chop the avocados and toss with the juice from half a lime.
6. Toast the pumpkin seeds in a dry pan briefly until slightly golden.
7. Top the potatoes with the avocado, then crumble over the cheese.
8. Sprinkle with the toasted seeds.

9. Serve and enjoy with lime wedges.

Lemon sole with chipotle and ancho chili recado

Ingredients

- 1 ripe avocado
- Extra virgin olive oil
- 2 limes
- 4 cloves of garlic
- 2 dried chipotle chilies
- 3 spring onions
- 2 dried ancho chilies
- 1½ tablespoon of dried oregano
- 4 lemon sole
- ½ a lime
- 14 ripe cherry tomatoes
- 1 Lebanese cucumber

Directions

1. Preheat the oven ready to 380°F.
2. Place the unpeeled garlic in a small roasting tin and roast for 20 minutes.
3. Transfer to a plate, let cool, then remove the skins.

4. Place the chipotle together with the ancho chilies in a small bowl.

5. Pour over boiling water to just cover, let soak for 15 minutes.

6. Drain in a colander, reserving some liquid.

7. Place the chilies together with the garlic, oregano, and a large pinch of sea salt in a food processor and blend to a paste.

8. Add the lime juice and 4 tablespoons of the reserved liquid, blend further to combine.

9. Transfer to a non-reactive bowl.

10. Place the fish in the marinade, cover with Clingfilm.

11. Refrigerate for 30 minutes.

12. Combine chopped cucumber, spring onions, tomatoes, an avocado in a bowl with 3 tablespoons of oil and the lime juice.

13. Season.

14. Preheat a barbecue to a medium heat.

15. Remove the fish from the refrigerator and cook, turning once, for about 3 minutes each side, brushing with marinade during cooking.

16. Serve and enjoy with the avocado salad and freshly squeezed lime wedges.

Salsa Verde fresco

Ingredients

- ½ a bunch of fresh coriander
- 2 large fresh green chilies
- 2 limes
- 12 green tomatillos
- 2 onions
- 1 ripe avocado
- 1 clove of garlic

Directions

1. Heat a griddle pan until screaming hot.
2. Then, chargrill the chilies until their skins are black and blistered all over.
3. Place the charred chilies in a bowl, cover with Clingfilm, let sit for a few minutes.
4. In batches, chargrill the tomatillos with onion wedges until blackened and caramelised on all sides.
5. Remove the chilies from the bowl and peel off the blackened skin.
6. Place the chilies together with the onions, garlic, tomatillos, coriander leaves, and avocado on a big board.

7. Chop all vegetables, mix in the lime juice and a good pinch of sea salt and black pepper.
8. Blend all the ingredients in a blender until smooth.
9. Drip onto eggs or on crispy chicken.
10. Serve and enjoy.

Chilled avocado soup with tortilla chips

Ingredients

- 1 handful of micro garlic chives
- ½ tablespoon of olive oil
- 1 cucumber
- 4 spring onions
- 200ml of plain yoghurt
- ½ teaspoon of hot smoked paprika
- A few sprigs of fresh coriander
- 2 soft corn tortillas
- 1 large ripe avocado
- 250ml of organic vegetable stock
- 1 mild fresh green chili
- 1 lime
- Tabasco sauce
- 1 fresh red chili

Directions

1. Preheat the oven to 400°F.
2. Combine the oil together with the paprika, brush over both sides of the tortillas.

3. Bake on a baking tray for 5 minutes, or until golden.
4. Season well and set aside to cool, break into pieces.
5. Blend the avocado together with the cucumber, stock, yoghurt, spring onions, coriander, and green chili until smooth.
6. Then, season with lime juice, Tabasco, and a good pinch of sea salt and black pepper.
7. Cover and place in the fridge to chill.
8. Once the soup is chilled, serve in small bowls topped with the tortilla chips, chopped cucumber, red chili and garlic chives.
9. Serve and enjoy with a drizzle of avocado oil.

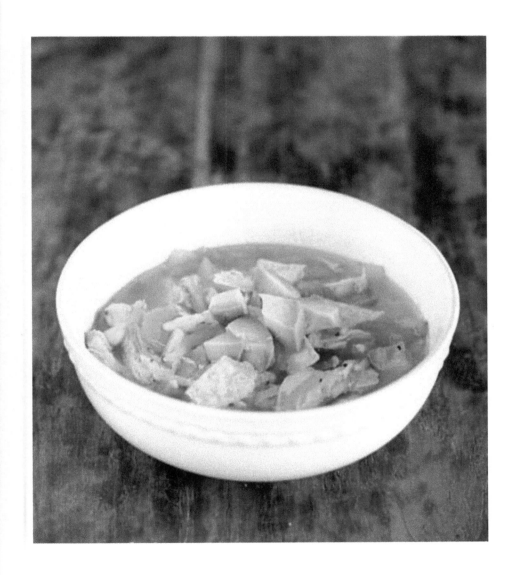

Lightning Source UK Ltd.
Milton Keynes UK
UKHW020748030621
384855UK00001B/110